CELLFOOD®

Vital Cellular Nutrition for the
New Millennium

By Dr. David S. Dyer

Important

The information in this book is intended for educational purposes only and is not recommended as a means of diagnosing or treating an illness. Nu Science Corporation, Division of Deutrel Industries, makes no medical claims or otherwise for the treatment, prevention, cure or mitigation of disease. Please consult a health practitioner for supervision of all matters concerning physical and mental health. Neither the publisher nor author directly or indirectly dispenses medical advice, nor do they prescribe any remedies or assume any responsibility for those who choose to treat themselves.

Acknowledgments

I would like to give acknowledgment to our Creator from whom I receive love, blessings, guidance and inspirations throughout my day. Without these wonderful gifts, my life would be empty and have little meaning. I am thankful for all that I have and for the opportunity to present this book to you. May the Creator bless you with love and understanding, for this is truly what the World needs more of.

On an Earthly plane I want to thank my daughter, Gentry. The presence of her sweet soul brings much joy into my life, and hope for her future. I pray she will take this information and use it to better her health and her life. Gentry, I am proud to be your dad and I love you with all that I have to give.

Table of Contents

Introduction

This book is a compendium of scientific facts as well as anecdotal information about CELLFOOD® and other important elements. I have arranged this information together in such a way that you can move through it quickly, gaining powerful knowledge. So much of the information available on the subject of natural health comes from the distant past. If you look at Hippocrates' teachings, you'll find an incredible amount of quality advice about living. After all, it was Hippocrates who said, "let your food be your medicine and medicine be your food." Many people refer to the Bible about eating and living habits: "be ye moderate in all things." It's great advice even today.

You see, everyone's health status today is a direct result of his or her lifestyle and eating habits of the past. If we want to improve our health we must change some things. Do you have to change everything today? No, but you must start somewhere. There is an old Chinese saying, "a journey of a thousand miles begins with the first step." I challenge you to take that first step. Another one that I like and use a lot is "yard-by-yard life is mighty hard, but inch-by-inch life is a cinch." These clichés are priceless analogies that can help us overcome the overwhelmed feeling we may experience when trying to make changes to improve our life.

My friend, this book and the information that it contains can be your first step towards better health and a happier life. Is it the final answer? No! Your body has additional requirements that will be covered in future publications. So, I challenge you to take this book and USE IT! Take back into your own hands the responsibility for your health. Regain the power that our Creator fully intended for you— and your loved ones— to have to live a healthier life. I am passionate about my health and the health of others. I wish you all good health…. because once you lose your health nothing else matters.

CHAPTER 1

CELLFOOD®: The Beginning

In order to tell the story of CELLFOOD®, let's begin with the background of the inventor Everett L. Storey. Albert Einstein called him a "genius," crediting him with the development of the "water-splitting" technology. He was truly an amazing man.

Although this extraordinary scientist is most remembered for his invention of the fusion trigger mechanism, Everett Storey's most significant achievements were designed to restore the environment and heal the human body. He was an expert in the little known uses of deuterium, the nonradioactive isotope of hydrogen — and knew all about the di-polar, di-base technologies using deuterium as their base. He was also knowledgeable about heavy water and atomic binding force technologies. During the second world war, Ev (as he preferred to be called) witnessed his discoveries being used to build the hydrogen bomb. But being a humanitarian, he wanted so much to do something *good* for humanity, and in the mid 1950's formulated a product that he named CELL-FOOD®— a nutritional supplementation product that he claimed could be the answer to any disease on earth. The same "water splitting" technology that was employed in the H-bomb's fusion trigger was incorporated into the CELLFOOD® technology. He thus created an oxygen therapy based on the ability of deuterium ions to self-sustain a catalytic type reaction in which our internal body water is dissociated into oxygen and hydrogen.

Everett Storey's proprietary CELLFOOD® formula is a result of 42 years of research (and in fact, it takes 9 months to create each batch!) Made from the finest plant substances, it's a formulation capable of holding its powerful elements in full solution and delivering them through ingestion to every single cell in the human body. This miraculous formula supports and enhances nutritional bio-chemical activities and brings to our diet what modern living and technologies have stripped away. Its constituent parts, including 78 trace elements and minerals, 34 enzymes, 17 amino acids, electrolytes— and nascent oxygen and hydrogen as byproducts— are all naturally occurring substances and essential to the body's many biochemical functions.

This is what Everett wrote in Beyond Belief, published by Feedback Books, Copyright 1982:

"Cellfood® dissociates water into nascent oxygen and hydrogen, and individual body cells are nourished by a steady stream of 78 essential elements maintained in free solution. This is due to the presence of free hydrogen and oxygen, which provides the oxidation and reduction in a chain reaction that eliminates toxins. Tissues are rebuilt, and then good nutrition completes the process.

Minerals are necessary for 95% of your body's daily functions. Minerals are life sustaining. Much of the natural trace mineral content has been lost from today's food supply due to depletion, poor crop rotation, loss of valuable topsoil due to flooding and over-irrigation."

Everett Storey's unique method of extracting and balancing nutrients in what he termed an "electromagnetic equation" will take contemporary scientists years to understand. Combining this equation with Storey's discovery of how to release oxygen and hydrogen from the tight polar bonding has resulted in the revolutionary CELLFOOD® products for treating the body, the skin and the environment.

Everett Storey's Biography

STOREY, EVERETT LAFAYETTE, publisher; born September 6, 1914; physical chemist; microbiologist; publisher; author; and football coach. Education: University of Chicago. Appts: Ed., Donnelley Advertiser, Chicago; owner, Canterbury Remembrancy Counselors, Chicago & NYC; Campaign Manager, Republican Party 17th Ward Chicago. Inventor: fusion trigger mechanism, 1942. Memberships include: Rushing Chairman, Sigma Chi; President, Southtown Speakers Club; Founder: Chicago Community Football League; American Medical Research Social & Academic; American Football; Coordinator, W. Alliance; Creative works include: publishing; producing & directing films; sculpture; painting; paper; American Chemical Society, Electroculture Cuts World Food Costs, 1976; perfected deuteron process, soil normalization that never stops.

•

Who's Who in the World
Marquis /Chicago 1978-79 Edition (page 896)

STOREY, EVERETT LAFAYETTE, publisher: b. Colorado Springs, Colo., Sept. 6, 1914, son of Walter Fletcher and Lois (DeLay) S.: ed. University of Chicago, 1932-36. Editor, Donnelley Advertiser, R.H. Donnelley Corp., Chicago., 1939-46; owner Canterbury Advertising Counselors, Chicago, N.Y.C., 1946-47; founder, publisher West Magazine Inc., Las Vegas, Nev. 1956-P, founder Deutrel Labs., Santa Paula Cal., 1965, controlling partner, 1966; president, Desert Reclamation Corp., Las Vegas, 1957-P, Executive secretary Long Beach Jr. Football League, 1949-49; executive director American Medical Research Society, 1959-63. Co-founder Shrimp Bowl, Chicago., 1948; chairman San Miguel Automated U. Study Group, Ventura, Cal., founder, head coach, Academy of

American Football, Santa Paula, Cal. Chairman Youth for Green, Ill., 1942-46. Chairman Republicans for Cannon, Nev. 1958. Recipient Community Service award Marshall Field, 1947, Member Sigma Chi. Club: Southtown Speakers (founder Chicago. 1938), Author: Getting Down to Fundamentals, 1943; 1966. Patentee fusion trigger mechanism; perfected deuteron process of soil normalization, 1960.

·

In addition to the above biographical information, Ev Storey was the author of the book "Beyond Belief," copyright 1982, published by Feedback Books. In this book he describes his life and beliefs in more detail. His discoveries with Deuterium and Tritium have opened up many new fields, including soil normalization, and reveal the potential future for Di-base solutions resulting from these discoveries. Covering more than 400 people and subjects, "Beyond Belief" is an education in itself. The Library of Congress Catalogue Card Number for this book is 82-70619.

CHAPTER 2

Oxygen, Hydrogen
& Other Essential Elements

Dr. Otto Warburg, renowned biochemist and 1931 Nobel Prize laureate, has shown that **cancer cells cannot grow in a high oxygen environment.** His lectures revealed that when oxidation fails and fermentation is substituted for a cell's energy, the pathway to cancer is opened. Dr. Warburg has said that: "The prime cause of cancer is the replacement of the normal oxygen respiration of body cells by an anaerobic (without oxygen) cell respiration." Dr. Warburg's discovery is just one of many compelling scientific facts which point to the vital importance of oxygen.

Oxygen is Life

Oxygen, carbon, hydrogen, nitrogen and sulfur are the five basic elements of all life. Of all the elements that support life, oxygen is the most abundant. Oxygen is essential for combustion (oxidation), and acts as a disinfectant, deodorizer, sanitizer and preserver. Oxygen makes up almost 50% of the earth's crust by weight, 42% of all vegetation, 85% of seawater, 46% of igneous rocks and 47% of dry soil. This colorless, tasteless and odorless element so essential to life comprises 65% of our body.

We can live a few days without water and a few weeks without food, but only a few minutes without oxygen. All functions of our body are regulated by oxygen. It must be replaced on a moment-to-moment basis because 90% of our life energy depends on it. Oxygen energizes cells so they can regenerate. Our body uses oxygen to metabolize food and to eliminate toxins and waste through oxidation. Our brain needs oxygen each second to process information. In fact, all of our organs need a great deal of oxygen to function efficiently. The ability to think, feel, move, eat, sleep and even talk all depends on generated energy from oxygen.

Oxygen is the only element capable of combining with almost every other element to form the essential components necessary to build and maintain our body. For instance, oxygen + nitrogen + carbon + hydrogen = proteins. Oxygen + carbon + hydrogen = carbohydrates. Oxygen + hydrogen = water. The combination of oxygen in the air, water, proteins and carbohydrates creates life energy. None of this energy could be produced without oxygen. As you can see, without oxygen we could not have the grand experience called life.

Oxygen and Health

Oxygen is one of five elements needed to sustain life— and clearly, one of the most important. For decades oxygen has been used to treat the sick and injured, and for the treatment of certain medical problems such as bone infections, wounds and other emergencies like carbon-monoxide poisoning and decompression sickness. (Only recently has the medical and sport professions begun to take a new and serious look at the value of increasing oxygen levels and the benefits that can be attained.)

Oxygen provides life and energy to every living cell. If poor eating habits, drinking, pollution, toxins, drugs or lack of exercise abuse the body, the cells are deprived of vital oxygen and the immune system may be weakened. Low oxygen levels are undesirable because they affect the body's cell metabolism and may even cause it to manufacture improper chemicals, and/or give rise to various health problems.

Though oxygen is one of the most important keys to good health, not everyone is aware of this. Scientists are only now looking at the important role that oxygen plays in the prevention of disease. The four modern-day stressors— toxic stress, emotional stress, physical trauma, and infections all draw upon and excessively deplete the body's oxygen supply.

Oxygen is absorbed by hemoglobin in the blood and is transferred to every cell in the body. Cellular homeostasis is dependent on adequate supply of oxygen in the blood. Life is indeed propelled by the oxygen in our blood— and a lack of oxygen results in sickness, poor vitality, poor stamina, fatigue and a general weak disposition.

Our normal level of oxygen reserves can be depleted over time by a number of factors including:

•**Toxic Stress**— toxic chemicals and air pollution, which are becoming more prevalent in our industrialized cities— as well as increased use of antibiotics;

•**Emotional Stress**— produces adrenaline and adrenal-related hormones, which utilize more oxygen;

•**Physical Trauma**— reduces circulation and oxygen supply to many cells and tissues throughout the body;

•**Infections**— use up "free radical" forms of oxygen to fight bacteria, fungi and viruses. Frequent use of drugs also depletes our oxygen supplies at the cellular level.

Research has shown that in most parts of the world the natural concentration levels of vital oxygen in our atmosphere are steadily decreasing due to climatic and industrial utilization changes that have taken place over the years.

Today, noted authorities also stress that most diseases, especially yeast or fungal infections like candida albicans, occur most frequently in any oxygen poor environment in the body. Dr. Stephen Levine, a molecular biologist and respected nutrition researcher, has also stated **"We can look at oxygen deficiency as the single greatest cause of all disease."** In his original hypothesis he has said that an "oxygen deficiency accompanies and is an integral aspect in all disease states." Thus the development of a shortage of oxygen in the blood could very well be the starting point for the loss of the immune system and the beginning of feared health problems such as cancer, leukemia, AIDS, seizures, nerve deterioration and candida.

If the normal environment of the cell can be maintained, it will not lose its growth and reproduction potential. Sub-oxygen creates sub-oxidation. An oxygen deficiency plays an important part in cellular contamination. Oxygen is a powerful detoxifier and when it is deficient, then toxins begin to devastate the body functions and deplete the body of life giving energy.

Oxygen Deficiency Symptoms

Initial symptoms of oxygen deficiency may include overall weakness, fatigue, circulation problems, poor digestion, muscle aches and pains, dizziness, depression, memory loss, irrational behavior, irritability, acid stomach, and bronchial complications. When the immune system is compromised by a lack of oxygen, the body is more susceptible to opportunistic bacteria, viral, and parasitic infections, colds, and flu. Oxygen deprivation can also trigger life-threatening diseases— as underscored by (twice) Nobel Laureate Dr. Otto Warburg's assertion that cancer and other infections or diseases cannot live in an oxygen-rich environment.

When scientists analyzed the oxygen content of air bubbles trapped in ice-core drillings in Antarctica, they found that the earth's atmosphere at one time contained between 38% and 50% oxygen. Over the years, increased pollution, increased toxins, mass rain forest destruction, and the reduction of other natural oxygen producers have decreased the level of oxygen in our present day atmosphere from these levels to below 20%. In overpopulated urban areas, the oxygen levels fall even lower. Because our bodies are not designed for low-level oxygen consumption, harmful toxins accumulate in our cells, tissues, organs, and bloodstreams. For comparative purposes, a 6% oxygen level causes human asphyxiation and death.

The industrial revolution, technological advancement and modern transportation have seriously depleted oxygen levels in our atmosphere. Our obsession with carbon-based fuels to power generators, planes and automobiles consumes vast amounts of oxygen daily. Coupled with this is the huge reduction of our forested areas and all plant life as the need for timber and paper continues beyond our production capacity. At the present time, research scientists have determined that our atmospheric oxygen concentration levels are being reduced by about 0.8% every 15 years or so. At the moment there is no reason to believe that this trend is going to change in the near future.

Knowledgeable scientists and doctors agree that the most common cause of metabolic disorders is oxygen-deficient blood. It is most recognizable by the creation of uric acid. This widely dispersed bodily poison is the basic cause of many chronic illnesses. The layman thinks of uric acid as a liquid. It may appear to be in solution, but as a rule it is in fact a fine crystal powder. Because of its insolubility, it is very dangerous. In order for the body to regain health, the body must be supported in its efforts to ingest sufficient oxygen to revitalize energy and cleanse itself of toxic substances.

Oxygen plays another very important role in the body, acting as a guardian and protector against unfriendly bacteria and disease organisms. One of oxygen's major functions is *disintegration*. Rubble, garbage, toxins, refuse, debris, and any useless substances are destroyed by oxygen and carried out of the system.

Oxygen Therapy

How important is oxygen to a healthy body? Many experts conclude that the lack of oxygen in human cells and tissue is linked to a vast variety of (and possibly all) health problems and disease, and that supplemental oxygen therapies have remarkable physiological benefits. A diversity of beneficial oxygen therapies are being utilized today.

What is oxygen therapy? Oxygen therapy is any supplemental process that safely increases the available dissolved oxygen content in the body. Therapies may also include processes that enhance the body's ability to use oxygen or promote oxygen absorption. Many of these oxygen therapy treatments are generally expensive, and should be administered or supervised by a licensed medical professional. Here are brief descriptions of some of the accepted oxygen therapies:

• **Bottled Oxygen**— is often prescribed as inhalation therapy for serious bronchial and other respiratory problems;

• **Ozone Therapy (O_3)**— generally infused rectally or intravenously, is primarily used to increase blood oxygenation, circulation, immunity, and to kill bacteria, viruses and fungi. The ozone oxygen molecule is extremely unstable and can be toxic if not administered properly;

•**Hydrogen Peroxide Therapy (H_2O_2)**— hydrogen peroxide is manufactured in the bloodstream to help fight bacteria, viruses, yeast, fungi, and other invading pathogens. The ingestion of H_2O_2 is extremely controversial because it can cause an adverse reaction in the digestive tract: excess hydrogen causes an unbalanced pH, as well as possibly producing dangerous free radicals. H_2O_2 therapy should only be utilized under the direct supervision of a licensed health care professional;

•**Breathing Exercises**— are thought to increase lung capacity, which transfers more oxygen to the bloodstream. Many people are shallow breathers, and disciplines such as yoga and other classes on diaphragmatic breathing can be very helpful;

•**Hyperbaric Oxygen Therapy (HBO)**— involves breathing oxygen in a pressurized chamber. This therapy saturates tissues and cells with oxygen, thereby greatly enhancing healing and immune-system response. HBO therapy was originally designed to treat divers and aviators for decompression sickness and air embolisms. Today HBO therapy is helpful in treating a wide variety of diseases, pathogens and degenerative conditions;

•**CELLFOOD® Dietary Supplement**— in my view, the easiest and most cost effective form of oxygen therapy is the daily ingestion of CELLFOOD®.

Hydrogen

Hydrogenation (also called reduction) is the addition of hydrogen to a molecule. Most body processes require hydrogen. Hydrogen plays a vital role in the *electron transport chain* (the route by which electrons transfer through a number of intermediate compounds that readily accept and release electrons, alternating between oxidized and a reduced form.) Fed by fusion and fission, hydrogen is the most common element in the universe. It builds cells and if left unmodulated, makes them hard and brittle. These affects are balanced by the action of oxygen.

Hydrogen is needed by the body to build and repair the immune system, the body's organs and cell structure. Everett Storey said, **"The winding road to health leads ever uphill from some form of hydrogen, probably Deuterium (its most versatile isotope) which is about to be recognized as the creative and sustaining force of all life."** Dr. Ev Storey utilized deuterium— which is used in the proprietary CELLFOOD® manufacturing process— to help hold the trace elements "in solution." This then enables the "water-splitting" technology to do its vital work.

The body normally obtains hydrogen from water, other liquids, fruits, and vegetables. A lack of hydrogen can lead to dehydration— causing extreme dryness and abnormal nerve heat generation inside the body. Because of dehydration, moisture and fatty nutrients are not well assimilated; this may result in brain shrinkage, face furrowing, drying of mucus, and tendon/nerve cramping. Other conditions caused by a lack of hydrogen include gout, muscular rheumatism, mental confusion and inadequacy, neck stiffness, irritated skin, and sore joints. Hydrogen, as well as oxygen, is released when CELLFOOD® is mixed with water— and continues releasing in a chain reaction for up to three days.

Water

In addition to oxygen and hydrogen, we need water to live. Unfortunately, the growing pollution in our modern day world is having an increasingly detrimental effect on our drinking water. Hazardous chemicals like mercury, lead, arsenic, cyanide, aluminum and phosphorus are getting into the water system every day. Other dangerous and toxic chemicals, including chlorine and fluoride, are added to reduce harmful microorganisms and prevent tooth problems. All these elements add to the load of toxins that our bodies have to eliminate.

For cleansing and nourishing our cells, research has proven that we need one-half our body's weight in fluid ounces per day (and more if we want to lose weight). This does not include coffee, teas, alcohol, fruit juices and other liquids. Dehydration causes bodily functions to go into distress, because fewer toxins are being removed, and less oxygen and nutrients can be transported throughout the body— especially to the brain, which is about 80% to 90% water. The remainder of the body is 70% to 90% water.

For good quality drinking water, we need to purify or filter the water before drinking it— and purified water is best for use with CELLFOOD®. Boiling water is not effective because although it kills the pathogens, it concentrates the pollutants that are in the water. There are many water purification systems to choose from today, as well as many types of bottled water using various purification processes— and this topic is so broad that it could be the subject of another book. CELLFOOD®, of course, is an extraordinary purifier of water and raises the frequency of water— however, I suggest that you start with the best quality water available to get the greatest benefits possible.

Minerals

From the dust of the Earth we were created. We therefore need, in proper quantities and proportions, over 70 minerals for peak performance of every cell in our body. But our soils are becoming more and more depleted of necessary minerals. Many fruits and vegetables now have less than 12 minerals out of the 70 plus that humans need for proper functioning— and which were present in our foods one hundred years ago.

We need minerals in our bodies for the proper composition of the body fluids, for the formation of blood and bone cells, and the maintenance of healthy nerve functioning. Lack of a single mineral in our food can cause mental and physical problems. We therefore need to become more aware of the nutritional value of each type of food, and eat the correct ones. We all know of the importance of calcium in our diets for building strong bones and teeth. However, because of the growing depletion of minerals in our foods, most of us probably also need some form of supplementation that will supply us with all the necessary minerals for the body's optimal performance.

"Do you know that most of us today are suffering from certain dangerous diet deficiencies which cannot he remedied until the depleted soils from which our foods come are brought into proper mineral balance? The alarming fact is that foods— fruits and vegetables and grains— now being raised on millions of acres of land that no longer contain enough of certain needed minerals, are starving us... no matter how much of them we eat!... Lacking vitamins, the system can make some use of minerals, but lacking minerals, vitamins are useless... A marked deficiency in any one

of the more important minerals actually results in disease... No man of today can eat enough fruits and vegetables to supply his stomach with the mineral salts he requires.... Our physical well-being is more directly dependent upon the minerals we take into our systems than upon calories or vitamins."

—Senate Document No. 264 (1936)

Strangely, all the talk about minerals today seems novel and quite startling. In fact the above information was readily available in 1936. A broadbased realization of the importance of minerals in food is so new that many textbooks on nutritional diets contain very little about it.

Nevertheless, it is something that concerns all of us, and is ever more pertinent today. The truth is that our foods vary enormously in value, and some of them just aren't worth eating as food. Our physical well-being is more directly dependent upon the minerals we take into our systems than upon calories or vitamins, or upon the precise proportions of starch, protein or carbohydrates we consume.

You'd think, wouldn't you, that a carrot is a carrot, that one carrot is about as good as another as far as nourishment is concerned? But it isn't; one carrot may look and taste like another and yet be lacking in the particular mineral element which our body system requires and which carrots are supposed to contain. Laboratory tests prove that the fruits, the vegetables, the grains, the eggs, and even the milk and the meats of today are not what they were a few generations ago (which explains why our forefathers thrived on a selection of foods that would now starve us!)

No longer does a balanced and fully nourishing diet consist merely of so many calories or certain vitamins or a fixed proportion of starches, proteins and carbohydrates. We know that our diets must contain minerals. I strongly suggest that one consume organic fruits and vegetables when available. Foods grown without chemical fertilizers, pesticides and herbicides taste different and better, and have a greater amount of naturally occurring vitamins and minerals. As mentioned before, the factory farmed foods of today are deficient in many nutrients that our bodies must have to achieve optimal health.

We know that vitamins are complex chemical substances needed for proper nutrition, and that each of them is important for normal function of many special structures in the body. Out of balance conditions and disease may result from vitamin deficiencies. It's not commonly realized, however, that vitamins control the body's appropriation of minerals, and in the absence of minerals they have no function to perform. Lacking vitamins, the system can use minerals, but lacking minerals, vitamins are useless.

Benefits of Trace Elements

Trace elements are minerals that the body requires in amounts of 100 mg or less, per day. For some, including iodine, proper dosage may be as small as one-tenth of 1 mg. Minuscule as these amounts are, insufficient intake of trace elements can seriously impair your health.

CELLFOOD® has 78 trace elements and minerals in its proprietary formulation; here, I've highlighted a few— and describe their specific importance:

•**Chromium (Cr)**— Enables the body to burn sugar, providing energy while preventing damage to blood vessels and organs. Natural sources: liver, brewer's yeast, black pepper, thyme, beef, poultry, broccoli, bran and whole grain cereals.

• **Copper (Cu)**— Necessary for the formation of blood cells and connective tissue. It is also involved in producing the skin pigment melanin. Natural sources: beef or chicken liver, crab, chocolate, seeds, nuts, fruit, and beans.

• **Iodine (I)**— Used by the thyroid gland to produce hormones essential for growth, reproduction, nerve and bone formation, and mental health. Natural sources: fish, shellfish, kelp and dulse.

• **Iron (Fe)**— Produces hemoglobin, the protein that carries oxygen throughout the body. It is also involved in the production of certain hormones, connective tissues and brain neurotransmitters, and immune system maintenance. Natural sources: liver, meat, poultry, fish, beans, nuts, dried fruits, whole grains, and dark leafy vegetables.

• **Manganese (Mn)**— Antioxidant; plays an important role in chemical reactions involving energy production, nerve-cell metabolism, muscle contraction, and bone growth. Natural sources: nuts, vegetables, and fruit.

• **Molybdenum (Mo)**— Antioxidant; helps the body remain healthy by detoxifying sulfites and sulfur compounds. Natural sources: milk, beans, bread, and cereals.

• **Selenium (Se)**— May help prevent some forms of cancer and heart disease. Also helps to boost the immune system. Natural sources: broccoli, mushrooms, cabbage, celery, cucumbers, onions, and garlic.

•**Zinc (Zn)**— Involved in the structure and function of all cell membranes as well as in production of more than 200 enzymes. Also is essential for proper wound healing. Natural sources: oysters, beef, pork liver, beef liver, lamb, crab, and wheat germ.

Metabolism and Enzymes

Metabolism is the sum of all chemical reactions in the living cell that are used for the production of useful work, and the synthesis of cell constituents. Almost all cellular reactions are catalyzed by complex protein molecules called enzymes, which are capable of speeding reaction rates by a factor of hundreds to millions. Most structures in the living cell are complex and require periodic replacement. This process of building new molecules is called *anabolism*. Structures that are no longer used are broken down into smaller molecules and either reused or excreted— this process is called *catabolism*.

Oxidation and Reduction

The vast majority of living organisms rely on oxygen to generate oxidative power. The actual mechanism is not a direct chemical reaction, but rather a series of *electron transfers* through a number of intermediate compounds that readily accept and release electrons alternating between an oxidized and reduced form. This route is called the electron transport chain and is similar in all organisms. As the strongest oxidizing agent of the chain, oxygen is the final electron acceptor. Oxygen's vital role in living organisms is essentially as a substance on which to "dump" electrons. (Many microorganisms are *anaerobic* and do not require oxygen for survival. These organisms are able to utilize sulfur and other compounds as oxidizing agents).

All organisms generate reducing power through the reversible biochemical reactions of nicotinamide-adenine dinucleotide (NAD), flavins, cytochromes, and other substances while existing in an oxidized or reduced form. By participating in the electron transport chain, the reduced form is continually regenerating from the oxidized form.

Enzymes

In order for the body to draw valuable nutrients from the food that we eat, it is necessary for the food to be properly digested and metabolized. Digestive enzymes do the work of digestion. *Amylase,* for example, breaks down carbohydrates. Metabolic enzymes then help to catalyze the various chemical reactions within the cells, such as energy production and detoxification—and in this way they assist in building the body from proteins, carbohydrates and fats. An example is *catalase,* which breaks down hydrogen peroxide in the body and liberates more oxygen for the body to use.

Unfortunately, once again, our modern life-styles are having a negative impact on these important enzymes. Enzymes are extremely sensitive to heat and are destroyed by temperatures above 50 degrees Celsius or 122 degrees Fahrenheit. Because we cook (and often over-cook) our foods, we need to eat more raw vegetables and fruits and supplement our intake of enzymes. CELL-FOOD® supplies 34 metabolic and digestive enzymes.

Amino Acids

Finally, in order for the body to use the food that we eat, the body needs amino acids to make up its necessary proteins.

Strangely enough, the proteins that the body uses are not obtained directly from the food we eat. Dietary protein is first broken down into amino acids, which the body then uses to build the specific proteins, hormones, antibodies and neurotransmitters it needs. CELLFOOD® supplies 17 amino acids to assist in these functions.

CHAPTER 3

The Anatomy of CELLFOOD®

CELLFOOD® is a highly-concentrated super-energized proprietary formulation containing 78 ionic/colloidal trace elements
and minerals (34 from fossilized plant taken from virgin earth,
and 44 from the clean Southern Seas surrounding New Zealand,
unrefined and still containing natural trace elements), combined
with 34 enzymes, 17 amino acids, dissolved oxygen— and all suspended in a solution of Deuterium Sulfate $[D_2 SO_4]$. As a complete mineral and nutritional supplement, CELLFOOD® enhances
nutritional biochemical activities and brings to your body what
modern living and technology are stripping away.

All the elements in CELLFOOD® are natural substances.
CELLFOOD® has no alcohol, no glucose, and no ingredients that
are on the 'list of banned substances' regarding international, professional and amateur athletic associations. The CELLFOOD® elements are derived from only the finest natural sources, which are
cryogenically (using extreme cold) and not chemically extracted—
and which are totally non-toxic.

The nutrients in CELLFOOD® are both ionic and colloidal
in form. Colloidal particles are minute (4-7 nanometers in diameter) and, because of the Brownian Movement Phenomenon, they
take on a negative (ionic) charge, and remain suspended in liquid.
Because most bodily fluids (like blood and lymph) are colloidal and
negatively charged, the body perceives CELLFOOD® as normal
healthy body fluid, and allows the nutrients in CELLFOOD® to
pass immediately through the sensitive membranes of the mouth,
throat and esophagus directly into the bloodstream.

CELLFOOD®'s Nutrients:

CELLFOOD® is made from only the finest natural plant substances. It's sourced from the clean southern seas surrounding New Zealand, from mineral springs and from fossilized plant taken from virgin earth.

1. Enhanced Oxygen

Oxygen is vital to the healthy functioning of our body— it fuels all of its systems, fires its chemical reactions, and eliminates wastes and toxins. CELLFOOD® enhances the bioavailability of oxygen to the body through its unique ability to 'dissociate' water molecules within the body— releasing abundant nascent oxygen and hydrogen directly to the cells.

2. Trace Elements and Minerals*

Actinium	Europium	Magnesium	Rhodium	Tungsten
Antimony	Fluorine	Manganese	Rubidium	Vanadium
Argon	Gadolinium	Molybdenum	Ruthenium	Xenon
Astatine	Gallium	Neodymium	Samarium	Ytterbium
Barium	Germanium	Neon	Selenium	Zinc
Beryllium	Gold	Nickel	Silica	Zirconium
Bismuth	Hafnium	Niobium	Silicon	
Boron	Helium	Nitrogen	Silver	***Note the**
Bromine	Holmium	Osmium	Sodium	**absence of**
Calcium	Hydrogen	Oxygen	Sulfur	**aluminum,**
Carbon	Indium	Palladium	Tantalum	**cadmium,**
Cerium	Iodine	Phosphorous	Technetium	**chlorine,**
Cesium	Iridium	Platinum	Tellurium	**mercury,**
Chromium	Iron	Polonium	Terbium	**lead, radium**
Cobalt	Krypton	Potassium	Thallium	
Copper	Lanthanum	Praseodymium	Thorium	
Dysprosium	Lithium	Promethium	Tin	
Erbium	Lutetium	Rhenium	Titanium	

3. Metabolic Enzymes

Hydrolases, Carbohydrases:
Maltase
Sucrase
Emulsin

Nucleases:
Polynucleotidase
Nucleotidase

Hydrases:
Fumarase
Enolase

Peptidases:
Aminopolypeptidase
Dipeptidase
Prolinase

Copper Enzymes:
Tyrosinase
Ascorbic Acid Oxidase

Esterases:
Lipase
Phosphotase
Sulfatase

Iron Enzymes:
Catalase
Cytochrome oxidase
Peroxidase

Enzymes containing coenzymes 1 and/or 2:
Lactic Dehydrogenase
Robison Ester Dehydrogenase

Yellow Enzymes:
Warburg's Yellow Enzymes
Diaphorase
Haas Enzyme
Cytochrome C reductase

Enzymes which reduce cytochrome:
Succinic Dehydrogenase

Amidase:
Urease

Mutases:
Aldehyde Mutase
Glyoxalase

Desmolases:
Zymohexase
Carboxylase

Other Enzymes:
Phosphorylase
Phosphohexisomerase
Hexokinase
Phosphoglumutase

4. Amino Acids

Alanine
Arginine
Aspartic Acid
Cystine
Glutamic Acid
Glycine
Histidine
Isoleucine
Lysine
Methionine
Phenylalanine
Proline
Serine
Threonine
Tryptophan
Tyrosine
Valine

5. Electrolytes

Electrolytes support the healthy electrical integrity of the body's natural colloidal systems, including the blood itself. They impart a negative charge to the red blood cells, separating them to restore their maximum functioning.

This highly efficient proprietary delivery system provides for over 95% bioavailablity (rapid, usable absorption at the cellular level) of CELLFOOD®'s 129 nutrients. This is very high, compared with the low absorption rates of tablets (25%) and gel caps (30%) — which have poor bioavailability because they're absorbed through the digestive system after various acids have broken them down. Furthermore, because CELLFOOD® is ionic/colloidal, the similarity between it and bodily fluids increases the bioavailability of nutrients in CELLFOOD® to every cell in the body. This increased availability of nutrients, and enhanced nutritional biochemical activity, enables the body to function optimally.

CELLFOOD® enables nascent oxygen to be generated by the splitting of water molecules in the body into atoms of nascent oxygen and hydrogen. Nascent means newly born; and, in biochemical terms, a newly born single atom of oxygen is negatively charged (O-). Free radicals (which many biochemists believe are the primary cause of premature aging and degenerative disease) are positively charged single atoms of oxygen (O+). The nascent oxygen atom (O-) is attracted to the (O+), forming a molecule of pure oxygen (O_2) at cellular levels where it is needed, for processes such as cleansing cells. Combined with a single carbon atom, it forms carbon dioxide (CO_2), which is expelled through the respiratory system.

Other Oxygen Products— and Free Radicals

Many oxygen products tend to flood the body with oxygen, often creating harmful oxygen free radicals. "The release of these reactive oxygen species results in oxidative injury to biologic systems such as lipids found in cell membranes, and proteins found in blood vessels and myocardial tissues." (Professors Ashim

Ghatak and Mahesh Chandra: Complementary Medicine, Page 13, Volume 4, Number 1, 1998).

CELLFOOD® has a more advanced technology, and it actually scavenges and bonds with dangerous oxygen free radicals, supplying the body with usable oxygen in a controlled and time-released manner at cellular level where it is needed. CELLFOOD®, therefore, does not create free radicals. It causes free radical single atoms of oxygen to be neutralized.

Another defense mechanism against free radicals is the enzyme *catalase*. "Catalase breaks down hydrogen peroxide, a metabolic waste product in the body, and liberates oxygen for the body to use." (James F Balch, M.D. & Phyllis A. Balch, C.N.C. Prescription for Nutritional Healing, Page 47, 1997). CELLFOOD® contains the enzyme catalase.

If people use other oxygen products, such as ozone and stabilized oxygenated water, they should use antioxidants to minimize the free radical effect that can be caused by the flooding effect of too much oxygen too quickly in the body. Obviously, CELLFOOD® would be ideal in this situation for normalizing and balancing the system.

The nascent hydrogen atoms created by CELLFOOD® are used by the body for many functions, such as irrigating, building and strengthening cells and organs; preventing inflammation, promoting osmosis, moistening lung surfaces for gas diffusion, and regulating body temperature. Hydrogen is essential for the processes of digestion, assimilation and elimination— and for transporting nutrients through the arteries to the brain and all body tissues. A person who weighs 175 lbs./80 kg. has about 15 lbs./7 kg. of hydrogen in his or her body.

When we speak of balancing a person, we refer to all the systems, including physical, electrical, biological, chemical, emotional, psychological and spiritual. CELLFOOD® is remarkable because it helps balance a person on almost all of these levels. CELLFOOD® works at the physical level by providing the body with essential minerals for the constitution of the physical body; it works at the electrical and electromagnetic levels by increasing the vibrational frequencies of all the body organs, boosting the immune system, and enabling the nervous system to function more effectively; it works at the biological level by enhancing natural biological processes, e.g. digestive and metabolic processes in the body (because of enzymatic action); and it works on the chemical level by supplying amino acids to the body for building protein. And CELLFOOD®'s ability to supply oxygen and nutrients to the brain supports emotional and psychological well-being.

How to Take CELLFOOD®

CELLFOOD® is a liquid concentrate. Mix 8 drops in an 8 oz. glass of purified water (if you use ordinary tap water, the CELLFOOD® starts purifying the water and the benefit you receive from the CELLFOOD® is reduced.) CELLFOOD® has a slightly sour lemon taste; taken with water or your favorite fruit juice it's quite good. Ev used to mix his in grape juice. Remember, CELLFOOD® contains natural, organic enzymes which are vital and powerful—and should be poured carefully in its non-diluted form, as it can mar clothing or organic surfaces (these enzymes enable CELLFOOD® to do its remarkable work.) Once diluted, CELLFOOD® is safe if spilled on any surface.

Everyone's body is different and each person has unique needs, and because CELLFOOD® is a nutritional supplement, each individual will respond in a unique manner. Optimal dosage is 8 drops three times a day. Many people take 12 drops first thing in the morning and 12 drops in the early evening instead. Some people, including athletes, mix a day's supply in a water bottle and sip it throughout the day. Initially CELLFOOD® may cause your body to begin a detoxification process. I will discuss the benefit of detox later in this chapter.

Start with the suggested dosage. Depending on how comfortable you feel with the response you are experiencing, you may then either reduce or increase the dosage. If you take less, the process of detoxification will slow down. If you take more, the process will accelerate. You also may simply feel a very pleasant feeling of increased energy and/or increased mental clarity.

If you experience no difference when taking 8 drops per dose, you can increase the dosage to 10, 12, or more drops, over a period of a few days until you experience a noticeable response. You cannot overdose on CELLFOOD®. Because it is a nutritional supplement made from natural substances, the body only uses what it needs, and eliminates the remainder through normal channels of elimination.

Some people take small doses three or more times a day to help them overcome a cold, or in times of distress. Take CELL-FOOD® as often as you particularly need it. Listen to your body's requirements, and take it when you sense that you need to. When feeling run down or stressed, take additional dosages. If you have to do some strenuous work, have a demanding sports activity, have to stay up late at night to work, have to drive somewhere or entertain guests, etc., take an extra dose of CELLFOOD® just beforehand to give your body additional energy.

Detoxification Information

When you first take CELLFOOD®, you may experience some noticeable form of detoxification, such as more frequent bowel movements and urination, slight nausea, mild headaches, and discharges. As the body receives a constant stream of the essential building blocks that it needs to strengthen its systems, it begins to clean house. The body starts to liquify accumulated waste and toxins that may have been lodged in the tissues, cells and organs of the body for many years, and to eliminate them in various forms such as phlegm and mucus.

If you do experience signs of detoxification, it's important to go through this process, which lasts from 1 - 3 days (sometimes longer,) because although you may feel slightly uncomfortable for a while, afterwards you will experience a new level of vitality. This process of detoxification can be called a "healing crisis," which is a sudden and acute reaction brought on by the strengthening of the body's energy or "chi," so that old toxins can be eliminated. Regular use of CELLFOOD® will assist the body to strengthen, and to eliminate more accumulated toxins.

I always tell people that CELLFOOD® may start some form of elimination of these old accumulated toxins. If, however, you feel unacceptably uncomfortable about this temporary process, then you should seek advice from a health practitioner who is knowledgeable about detoxification processes. It's unfortunate when someone stops taking CELLFOOD® because they were not prepared to go through some level of cleansing.

Hering's Law of Cure and Retracing

Knowing Hering's Law of Cure can help you to continue your detoxification process; it is very important in understanding the difference between "healing" and "disease." The famous homeopath, Constantine Hering, made a clear distinction between the symptoms of a disease crisis and those of a healing crisis. Unfortunately, due to ignorance, we confuse a healing process with a disease process and suppress it with medication. This only makes the body weaker and more susceptible to disease.

Hering's Law of Cure states: "All cure starts from the head down, from within, out, and in the reverse order that the symptoms appeared throughout the person's life."

When a person experiences a healing crisis, it is essential to give this process assistance in order to promote the elimination of toxins and disease elements that may be manifesting themselves as phlegm, catarrh, mucus, runny nasal discharge, enlarged tonsils, fever, etc. This is nature's way of righting some internal wrong; it is also known as "retracing." Whatever has been suppressed in the body for years (e.g. some childhood illness that was suppressed with medication) liquifies and is removed through normal elimination channels. As the body's health improves you may, unexpectedly, experience another cleansing. You may go through a number of healing crises over a period of time. Each time, stored toxins are eliminated; you may experience new levels of vitality and health. Sometimes a person is unaware of the process that CELLFOOD® is facilitating at deep cellular levels. Because of this you may not be consciously aware of what is happening; you may think that CELLFOOD® is not working for you. Some individuals have had no noticeable results at first from taking CELLFOOD®, but later, after having undergone regular medical check-ups, reported that their cholesterol and blood pressure levels had dropped significantly. There are similar accounts regarding the normalization of uric acid and blood-sugar levels. In other cases CELLFOOD® has worked at deep cellular levels, improving

Comparison between a Disease Crisis and a Healing Crisis:

Disease Crisis	Healing Crisis
1. Can start gradually and is developed over a period days. In most cases, it can be for months and years.	1. Starts suddenly, after feelings of perfect health.
2. Results from abuse, improper living and eating habits, over-use of medications etc.	2. Results from a prescribed healthy program, or starts spontaneously, sometimes after stopping medications.
3. Lasts usually more than 3 days.	3. Lasts usually about 1 - 3 days (sometimes longer).
4. Inefficient or lacking elimination.	4. Proper elimination.
5. Usually the symptoms are different from any previously experienced.	5. Repeating of old symptoms in a reverse order to the appearance of the "disease crises" throughout one's life.
6. After the crisis, there is usually a period of convalescence.	6. After the crisis, the condition improves very quickly.
7. Damaged tissue does not regenerate, or regenerates partially over a period time.	7. Damaged tissue almost always regenerates after a few weeks or months.
8. The doctor can relieve or aggravate the crisis, usually by using medication (to suppress the crisis).	8. The individual should do nothing to alleviate the crisis. They should contact a health consultant and adviser for guidance.
9. The events of the crisis are different and unpredictable each time; after the crisis, the person feels worse, or the same as they felt before the crisis.	9. The events of the crisis are definitive, according to Hering's Law of Cure: and after the crisis the person feels years younger with lots of energy.
10. A person can die in a disease crisis.	10. A healing crisis never ends in death!

the immune system. In addition to assisting with the cleansing of cells, CELLFOOD® increases the vibrational frequency of all organs, making them more resistant to lower-frequency viruses, bacteria and parasites.

Once again, it is important to realize that CELLFOOD® itself is not directly curing disease. The body has been magnificently designed by Our Creator to do that. CELLFOOD® is amazing because it provides the cells with essential building blocks needed to perform required normal functions to achieve optimal health. Because CELLFOOD® works in a natural way at normalizing and balancing the body, I always encourage users to continue taking CELLFOOD®, and become more attentive to the less noticeable but more significant changes in their bodies. A sure way of becoming aware of what CELLFOOD® is achieving is to examine the comparative results of medical exams before and after the use of CELLFOOD®. This gives clear evidence that CELLFOOD® has been normalizing and balancing all bodily systems, and facilitating renewal at deep cellular levels.

Though I often explain that CELLFOOD® works on priorities at deep cellular levels— and works wonders at normalizing and balancing many of our systems— some people may not experience the results they desire. In these cases I ask the following:

1) **Where do you store your bottle of CELLFOOD®?** Some people have stored the bottle on a microwave oven or in a handbag near a cellular phone. In these cases the electrical fields may have reduced the effectiveness of CELLFOOD®. Generally, nutritional supplements should be kept away from such appliances.

2) **How do you take CELLFOOD®?** For best results, CELLFOOD® should be taken with purified water or juice, separate from meals. Allow at least 15-20 minutes before eating, or at least 45 minutes after a meal.

3) **How much and how often are you taking CELLFOOD®?**
Recommended dosage is 8 drops 3 times per day. If you have no apparent benefit you may increase the amount. As previously explained, CELLFOOD® is working at some level in the body that may not be apparent to the user; and, because of the small dosage, there is not enough in your particular system for work to take place. I suggest that you increase the dosage (e.g. an extra 2 or 3 drops every 3 days) until benefits are noticed. At a later stage, reduce the dosage to a maintenance level of 8 drops 3 times a day.

Finally, I suggest that you should simply stop taking the CELLFOOD®, and notice how you feel. Often, when a person suddenly stops taking CELLFOOD®, they then become aware of how it had been incrementally assisting them with more energy and alertness, etc. If someone experiences no detoxification after taking CELLFOOD® it may be that their body isn't in need of detox at that particular time. They may experience these conditions later. I recommend doing a specific detox program at least twice a year.

During a healing crisis, you may feel that you lack energy. This is probably because your body is cleansing, restoring, etc. at deep cellular levels, and is using a lot of energy for this. By continuing to take CELLFOOD® and drinking lots of liquids, you will assist the body to go through the healing crisis. After the healing crisis (usually from 1 to 3 days), you will feel more energetic than you have felt for years. If the healing crisis persists for more than 1 week, consult with a health practitioner who is experienced in the processes of detoxification and healing crises.

CELLFOOD® is not a medicine, and no medical claims are made for the treatment, prevention, cure or mitigation of disease. Therefore there are no published clinical tests, as is the case with medicines. With medicine, there is a cause and effect relationship, so Medicine A will produce Effect B, and clinical tests can prove this. Because CELLFOOD® is a nutritional supplement it works with the body's priorities, and starts working where it is most needed. Therefore, because everyone is unique, we cannot prove that CELLFOOD® does any specific thing. We can, however, tell people about other people's experiences, and there are thousands of testimonials worldwide.

Therefore, I never make any medical claims about CELL-FOOD®, so that I am not in violation of the present regulations of any governing agency. Hopefully, one day CELLFOOD® may be positioned in its rightful place as one of the most incredibly advanced developments for cleansing, repairing, building, balancing and energizing the human body.

When the "water splitting phenomenon" takes place, the nascent hydrogen atoms contain enormous supplies of positively charged electromagnetic energy. One drop of CELLFOOD® produces 77,000 angstroms of energy. This hydrogen energizes the body. In 1991, Dr. Aristo Vojdani, V.P. of lmmunosciences Laboratories Inc. U.S.A. reported "significant increases in T-cells with increasing dosages of CELLFOOD®." This means that as the immune system is being progressively boosted, it makes the body more capable of dealing with microorganisms that could be detrimental to one's health.

"I think what the man in the street wants to know is how CELLFOOD® will react on their different diseases. That's what I find is the most important thing. They phone me every day and tell me what they've got. It doesn't matter what type of disease the person has, it's that the additional oxygen in the bloodstream with the hydrogen molecules is definitely going to bond in a better format to create a better cell." (**Dr. Linet Stockdale**, Hematologist; South Africa.)

"Cancer, above all other diseases, has countless secondary causes, but there is only one prime cause... The prime cause of cancer is the replacement of the normal oxygen respiration of body cells by an anaerobic cell respiration." (**Dr. Otto Warburg**, two-time Nobel Laureate Winner of the Nobel Prize for Cancer Research.)

"Since Warburg's discovery, this difference in respiration has remained the most fundamental (and some say, only) physiological difference consistently found between normal cells and cancer cells. Using cell culture studies, I decided to examine the differential responses of normal and cancer cells to changes in the oxygen environment. The results that I found were rather remarkable. I found that "normal" O_2 tension actually maximized the growth of the cancer tissue, and that high O_2 tensions were lethal to cancer tissue, 95 percent being very toxic, whereas in general, normal tissues were not harmed by high oxygen tensions. Indeed, some normal tissues were found to require high O_2 tensions. It does seem to demonstrate the possibility that if the O_2 tensions in cancer tissues can be elevated, then the cancer tissue may be able to be killed selectively, as it seems that the cancer cells are incapable of handling the O_2 in a high O_2 environment." (**J. B. Kizer:** Biochemist and Physicist, Gungnir Research, Portsmith, OH.)

As CELLFOOD® has become better known for supplying the body with the building blocks it needs to improve our quality of life, many people in government, business, sport, etc. are benefiting by taking CELLFOOD®. Professional and amateur athletes "testing" CELLFOOD® report they feel more alert, excel at their particular sport (e.g. tennis, basketball, golf— as well as running, swimming, weightlifting, etc.) are less out of breath, recover more quickly after sport (CELLFOOD® cleanses the muscles of lactic acid), generally feel more positive and enjoy increased stamina.

On the other end of the health spectrum, those who do not eat properly, and who smoke and drink alcohol excessively, do not exercise, have no get-up-and-go in the morning, always feel tired and run down, can't get a good night's sleep, want more vitality and energy— and generally want more out of life— would greatly benefit by taking CELLFOOD®. With more oxygen and minerals in their systems, children, students, teachers, and workers have reported that the increase in their alertness level and attention span, as well as their ability to deal with stress and pressure, have amazed them.

Many doctors are advising their patients to take CELL-FOOD® as supplementation to other medications, remedies or supplements they may be taking. CELLFOOD® makes the other preparations more bio-available in the body. There are thousands of testimonials worldwide about the benefits of taking CELL-FOOD®. People who seem to have an immediate response from using CELLFOOD® are those who have been suffering from arthritis and other degenerative diseases. Some have reported the disappearance of pain from their joints within a few days of taking CELLFOOD®, and later reported that their swollen joints were gradually reducing in size.

Other people report that a cold stays only for a day or two compared to previously, when it would linger for over a week. Remember, CELLFOOD® is not a medicine; it merely provides the body with all the building blocks in order for it to function optimally. Because this often results in a stronger immune system, a previously sick person now has the strength to fight a disease, and can begin to heal. I cannot claim that CELLFOOD® cured the person. It initiated a process, and assisted the body to strengthen his or her immune system in order to fight and defeat the disease.

CELLFOOD® can be used in conjunction with other nutritional supplements or medicines, because it increases the bioavailability of other substances so that they may be more effectively utilized by the body. That's why people who are on heavy medication and who take CELLFOOD® must be regularly monitored by their health practitioners. Within a few weeks or months the need for medication can often be gradually decreased as the body cleanses, gets stronger and more balanced. The decrease of medication should be done only under the direction of their doctor.

CELLFOOD® can be applied externally on the skin; either undiluted (using a Q-tip) on warts, moles, small growths, burns, etc., or diluted 1:10 parts distilled water for skin rashes, 1:20 parts distilled water on open wounds, 1:30 parts distilled water for sinus and ear problems, and 1:60 parts distilled water for eye infections.

There are many reported cases of animals benefiting from CELLFOOD®. Everett Storey himself put a couple of drops of CELLFOOD® into the bowl of water for his dogs. He withdrew all other sources of water. He did this for four days. Thereafter, he supplied his dogs with two bowls of water, one with CELLFOOD® and one without. The dogs always went to the bowl with CELL-FOOD® added, and lived very healthy lives.

By taking CELLFOOD® regularly, you are providing your body with the essential building blocks for the daily cleansing, nourishing, restoring, building and balancing of your body. In this way, you are making a meaningful investment in yourself; ensuring quick healing if you do get ill or injured; and improving your quality of life at every level.

In January 1978, Everett Storey applied for F.D.A. registration of "CELLFOOD®" (also known as Deutrosulfazyme). On the Pharmaceutical Composite Form he described it as: "Champagne color to amber color with passage of time, but instead of a loss in potency, there is actually a small increase each year."

Under the section "Therapeutic Effects", he stated that CELLFOOD®:

• Aids materially in the digestive process

• Assists in the cleansing of upper and lower intestines, and restores normal bowel functions.

• Enables the blood stream to deliver directly to each body cell a minimum of 78 assimilable elements for complete, direct and quick nutrition.

• Provides a steady flow of both oxygen and hydrogen to all parts of the body, thus effecting the hitherto "impossible achievement of simultaneous oxidation and reduction within a given cell."

In 1985 the American Government passed the "DEU-TERIUM FREEDOM ACT OF 1985" in which recognition was given to the amazing work of Everett Storey and his product, CELLFOOD®, (registered as Deutrosulfazyme by the American Department of Health in 1978 when Storey applied for registration with the F.D.A.)

The ACT, Section 2(b) Line 15 states: "Deuterium can and does form all other elements, and stands at the very core of the Universe. The ashes of hydrogen constitute water. Heavy Hydrogen combined with water becomes 'Heavy Water' (Deuterium Oxide). Line 25 states: "Because of Deuterium's facility to speed up the digestive process, it will aid in patients getting more mileage out of the food they consume; and, at the same time, reduce the toxicity in the blood stream. Deutrosulfazyme is a systemic normalizer. No wonder it is called Cellfood®.

International Recognition of CELLFOOD®

In 1997, CELLFOOD® was unanimously voted by the Inventors Clubs of America to receive the 1997 Advanced Technology Award presented by the International Hall of Fame in Atlanta, GA. CELLFOOD® received this award because of (1) its unique ability to produce both nascent oxygen and hydrogen inside the body, resulting in the simultaneous cleansing and building of body cells and tissues, and (2) its unique ability to maintain 78 elements, trace minerals and minerals in liquid colloidal suspension.

Research in Japan

In 1997, the Japanese Ministry of Health approved the sale of CELLFOOD® as a nutritional supplement. Apetie Link Company Limited in Japan tested the effect of CELLFOOD® on the average person's physical and mental areas, as well as its effect on vitality levels, and its ability to deal with disease conditions. For this purpose, they used the Magnetic Resonance Analyzer, an analyzing machine, developed in the U.S.A. for measuring frequencies and wave motion. It is now being used in more and more American and Japanese hospitals to diagnose the physical and mental conditions of patients. In Germany, they use a similar diagnostic machine, called the Vagar Analyzer.

Mr. Kohei Fukuda reported: "We tested CELLFOOD® with the Magnetic Resonance Analyzer (M.R.A.) and obtained results that are unbelievable. According to the results, CELLFOOD® is an incredibly good product. The M.R.A. measures up to a limit of +20. Some of the readings for CELLFOOD® *exceeded* this limit, which is incredible."

Items tested (in no particular order), code numbers, and measuring ratios are shown in the table that follows:

Item	Code	Ratio	Item	Code	Ratio
Natural healing power	2BD6	+20	Gall bladder	3423	+19
Circulation of blood	3CB7	+19	Heart	3423	+20
Environmental stress	3AA1	+16	Small intestine	368E	+18
Active oxygen	38BB	+16	Spleen	34E8	+19
Essential energy	3855	+20	Stomach	338F	+20
Mental energy	3411	+17	Lungs	36AC	+10
Communication	3830	+14	Large intestine	3365	+16
Self-confidence	3F9	+16	Kidneys	35BA	+18
Emotional energy	30F7	+17	Bladder	36FD	+7
Integration power	33F6	+18	Cervical vertebrae	389E	+6
Basic energy	3481	+19	Chest vertebrae	3GDE	+9
Intuition	32F1	+17	Lumbar	3619	+11
Thinking and I option	321A	+19	Cancer	3A9D	+20
Memory	3425	+18	Diabetes	35DD	+19
Volition	31E4	+17	Eczema	3E2F	+16
Autonomic nervous sys.	30F8	+18	Exhaustion	35AF	+18
Dealing with Anger	3568	+16	Pain	3432	+5
Dealing with Fear	3681	+8	Insomnia	3432	+16
Liver	3D9	+19	Mental unhealth	3A22	+12

This report clearly shows that CELLFOOD® is a very balanced product, and works on many levels in the body at the same time. We publish these findings because it is important for people to know how amazing CELLFOOD® is. Remember, CELLFOOD® is not a medicine; it is not intended for the treatment, prevention, cure or mitigation of disease. CELLFOOD® achieves results by providing the body with many of the building blocks that the body needs, in order for it to function optimally.

The shelf life of CELLFOOD® is indefinite; and when 25-year-old samples were tested, they showed an *improvement* in the potency of the product. CELLFOOD® is indeed prepared with an amazing formulation, and although attempts to duplicate it have been made none have been successful.

This formula is not patented; it is a proprietary (secret) formula and only two copies of the formula are in existence. Both are in safe places. I don't see the wonderful testimonials from any of the CELLFOOD® imitators that I see with CELLFOOD®, so be sure and use the original formula.

CELLFOOD® is manufactured by Nu Science Corporation, a division of Deutrel Industries. Duetrel Industries is licensed by the California Department of Health Services, Food and Drug Division. CELLFOOD® is available from various distributors, doctors, pharmacies and health food stores.

CHAPTER 4

CELLFOOD® FAQ (Frequently Asked Questions) and Testimonials

1. **Is CELLFOOD® a medicine?** **Answer:** No, CELLFOOD® is not a medicine. CELLFOOD® is classified as a nutritional supplement.

2. **What is the shelf life of CELLFOOD®?** **Answer:** The shelf life is indefinite. Recent testing of 25-year-old samples has demonstrated an improvement in potency.

3. **How does the body absorb CELLFOOD®?** **Answer:** The nutrients in CELLFOOD® are in colloidal/ionic form. Colloidal particles are minute (4-7 nanometers in diameter), and because of the Brownian Movement Phenomenon, they take on a negative (ionic) charge and remain suspended in liquid. Because most bodily fluids are colloidal and negatively charged, the body perceives CELL-FOOD® as normal healthy body fluid and allows the nutrients to pass immediately through the sensitive membranes of the mouth, throat, and esophagus directly into the blood stream.

4. **How does it work?** **Answer:** CELLFOOD® enables nascent oxygen to be generated by the splitting of water molecules in the body into atoms of nascent oxygen and hydrogen. In biochemical terms, a newly born single atom of oxygen is negatively charged (O-). Free radicals (which many biochemists believe are the primary cause of the aging process and degenerative disease) are positively charged single atoms of oxygen (O+). The nascent oxygen atom (O-) is attracted to the (O+) forming a molecule of pure oxygen (O_2) at the cellular level where it is needed.

5. How is CELLFOOD® different from other so-called oxygen products? Answer: Many other oxygen products tend to flood the body with oxygen, often creating dangerous oxygen free radicals. "The release of these reactive oxygen species results in oxidative injury to biologic systems such as lipids found in cell membranes, and proteins found in blood vessels and myocardial tissues." (Professors Ashim Ghatak and Mahesh Chandra: Complementary Medicine, p. 13, vol. 4, no. 1, 1998.) CELLFOOD® actually bonds with dangerous oxygen free radicals, supplying the body with usable pure oxygen, in a time-release manner, directly to the cells.

6. How do I take CELLFOOD®? Answer: CELLFOOD® is a liquid concentrate, taken orally by mixing a number of drops (see individual label for instructions) in purified water. If you use ordinary tap water, CELLFOOD® begins purifying the water and the benefit you receive from CELLFOOD® is reduced. CELLFOOD® has a slightly sour lemon taste which most people enjoy; taken with water or your favorite fruit juice it's quite good.

7. Can I overdose on CELLFOOD®? Answer: No, CELLFOOD® is a nutritional supplement made from natural substances. The body only uses what it needs, and eliminates the remainder through the normal channels of elimination.

8. What happens if I don't receive results? Answer: Sometimes a person is unaware of the "work" that CELLFOOD® is facilitating at deep cellular levels. People who first reported no results from taking CELLFOOD® later reported, after physical examinations, that their cholesterol and blood pressure levels had dropped significantly. There are similar accounts regarding the normalization of uric acid and blood sugar levels. Additionally, CELLFOOD® is designed to raise the frequencies of all organs, making them more resistant to the lower frequencies of viruses, bacteria, and parasites. This strengthening of the immune system helps the body become more capable of combatting microorganisms that could be detrimental to your general health.

9. Am I "cheating" if I use CELLFOOD® during sports competitions?   **Answer:** No, CELLFOOD® is made from the finest natural ingredients, none of which are on the "list of banned substances" issued and governed by professional and amateur athletic associations.

10. What if I am already taking medicine? **Answer:** CELLFOOD® can be used in conjunction with other nutritional supplements or medicines because it increases the bioavailability of these other substances, enabling the body to more effectively use them. Many CELLFOOD® users have reported a gradual decrease in need for medication within a few weeks or months of continual use (of CELLFOOD®). If you are pregnant or under medical care, please consult your medical practitioner before using.

Testimonials From CELLFOOD® users:

"Until recently I was a severe asthmatic suffering also from emphysema and chronic bronchitis, which originated from fighting a forest fire while serving in the U.S. Air Force. My condition over the years was gradually getting worse to the extent that for the past several months I was using 5 rescue inhalers every 90 days as well as 2 other stabilizing inhalers.

The first of January this year, I received my allotted medications and by the end of the month my condition had worsened to the extent that I was waking every 1-1/2 to 2 hours every night unable to breathe. During the day I was constantly sucking on an inhaler, as it seemed that I was perpetually short of breath.

I was introduced to CELLFOOD® the first part of February and started taking it right away. When I went in for my regular check- up on March third, the doctor was in awe when she noted that there was no railing or wheezing in my chest and that I was breathing with no shortness of breath.

I went in for a scheduled breathing test on the 24th of March. Oxygen content prior to this date was 60%, which is average for an asthmatic. This time it was 70%, a marked increase. The SD breathing had increased from 350 to 415. Quite an improvement. To this day, I have not been short of breath and have not taken any medication, but I am still taking CELLFOOD®."

MF— Oklahoma

"For a period of five years I have suffered from chronic back pain accompanied by fatigue. I have tried many innovative therapies, including both traditional and alternative modes of treatment for this disease. These treatments included drugs and physical therapy, a variety of nutritional therapies, acupuncture, neural therapy, radionics and massage. It was through the use of CELLFOOD® that I first obtained significant relief from the fatigue that interfered with my life. My day was comprised of work, then home to rest and sleep. The weekend was also spent resting.

I took CELLFOOD® on a regular three-times-daily basis, which refreshed and energized me. After three to four months of regular use I stopped using CELLFOOD®, only to find that the fatigue returned. Now that I'm back on the CELLFOOD® on a consistent basis, my energy has been restored. Research on CELLFOOD® indicates that it is a powerful electrolyte solution, that it works to energize the body and bring it into chemical and electrical balance. I find that I get a quicker and more complete therapeutic response to treatment when I prime my patients— especially the more difficult pain cases— with CELLFOOD®, prior to treating them with acupuncture and magnet therapy."

BBM, M.D.— Carmichael, CA

"CELLFOOD® is, in my estimation, the single item that can do more things than any other single item that I've been exposed to in 30 years of practice. What does it do? And what is it? It's a combination of a myriad number of natural elements, some from the sea, some from the earth. Those elements have been put together in such a way that they somehow have the potential to generate life. When these materials are ingested they provide a broad spectrum of highly energized elements that provide the body with what it needs to operate normally and for the construction of life. The way they are put together makes them accessible as highly charged bullets of chemistry. Positive things start to happen within the body— and the body begins performing, correcting its own problems, whatever they may be. That's CELLFOOD®. Dynamite! Drop by drop. Pearls of great wisdom for this body.

Because they are so potent, so energized, they can be used to potentiate any other substance you take— especially nutrients— to give you maximum potential and benefit. I couldn't believe, and I still hardly believe, that it works as well as it does, but it does!"

Dr. H, M.D.

"In recovering from a car accident, emotional trauma, cancer and more, CELLFOOD® made an immediate difference in my ability to cope with emotional trauma. My low energy has begun to improve. I'm experiencing some kind of intestinal cleansing with diarrhea over 4 days, interspersed with normal bowel movements."

Dr. G— Health Practitioner

"CELLFOOD® has helped clear up my skin and I have more energy, more endurance on the Stairmaster. I noticed results within three days."

Dr. C— Licensed Acupuncturist

"I've been in practice as an M.D. for 25 years— and a serious student of nutrition for several decades. In all these years I've never seen anything that even remotely compares to Cellfood as an overall benefit to the human body.

Aside from its great value taken internally, I personally utilized a topical solution made of a ratio of 1 drop of Cellfood to 10 drops of water, and— in 3 to 4 days— successfully treated my own eczema condition which I'd had for many years."

Dr. RN, M.D.— Hays, KS

"This is a letter of testimony about CELLFOOD®. I was very ill for 3 years with pneumonia, and was in and out of the hospital 3 times. Each time I was getting weaker and weaker. There was scar tissue on my lungs, causing irregular breathing patterns.

I was out of breath walking, climbing steps, had blackouts, and was unable to stand up very long. I work in a nutrition store in Ft. Lauderdale, so I have familiarity with nutritional products. We ordered some bottles of CELLFOOD®. I began using the product. To my surprise, within a week I was walking and standing up longer periods of time. Now I can walk up steps, without being out of breath. My doctor said I amazed her. My lungs were clear, and she could find nothing wrong with me. I walked 3 miles recently, and haven't walked that far in years. May God bless you for a magnificent product. I haven't felt this good in years!"

KCN— Ft. Lauderdale, FL

"All my life I've had to endure living with asthma. Anyone who has had a hard time breathing may think they know that being short of breath is uncomfortable, but they can't imagine what it is like to fight for the smallest gasp of air— while everything turns gray as your brain starves for oxygen. I know that feeling. I've been so dizzy and so close to passing out during a full phase asthma attack— all the fight leaves you, and you feel as if you could just let go and stop struggling. The next day, after a major attack, it feels as if my lungs and ribs got hit by a sledge hammer; I'm wiped out— just exhausted. I hate having asthma, and hate asthma medication.

Since taking CELLFOOD®, for the first time in my entire life I know what it feels like to take a deep, complete, satisfying lung full of air. Breathing is so much easier, and I can actually emerge from an attack much faster and easier. I don't struggle any more for every breath, every day. I am so grateful for this product. It has changed my life very much for the better."

LD— Apple Valley, CA

"I want to share my experience with CELLFOOD® after taking it 3 times daily for one month. I feel less stressed and more calm and relaxed— but most important to me is the effect on my blood pressure, which had been 150/90. Now my blood pressure fluctuates between 132/70 and 122/70. I'm one happy customer."

PJ— San Diego, CA

"I'm writing this testimonial simply to let you know how helpful CELLFOOD® has been to me. I have been diagnosed with HIV illnesss for about ten years now. Taking the CELLFOOD® has greatly increased my stamina and general energy level. In the past I had to take several naps per day, but since I've been on this wonderful product, I've felt no need to take these naps. I am able to carry on a full, active day, which was impossible 2 months ago.

I've also noticed that I sleep much better. I am more alert and better able to concentrate. As a Registered Nurse I am amazed with the effects that CELLFOOD® has produced in my life.

In closing, I would like to thank you for making this product available to myself and to anyone who may have similar challenges. CELLFOOD® has improved my quality of life substantially."

EG, R.N.— San Diego, CA

"Thank you for your wonderful CELLFOOD® product. I have had extreme pain from arthritis for years, and I have been afflicted with a seizure disorder since childhood. Until recently, I've been taking six to eight 600 mg. tablets of ibuprofen for pain, and also was taking seizure medication that was so strong that it created a mental fog similar to what one would experience taking a very strong antihistamine.

Since taking the CELLFOOD®, I no longer take any medication or pain killers, and for all practical purposes am seizure free. I'm simply adding CELLFOOD® in every glass of water I drink.

I also have more clarity of thought and more enegy. I now require less sleep— but awake refreshed and ready to start another pain and seizure-free day. I have my life back. Thank you!"

MP—San Diego, CA

"When a friend first told me about CELLFOOD$^®$, he told me to order at least three bottles— so I could put one next to my bottled water to add whenever I have a glass of water, one in the kitchen next to the stove in case I burn myself, and one to carry with me whenever I left the house. I'm glad I took his advice.

On Thanksgiving day, I was cooking a traditional dinner with lots of dishes. In the hecticness, I grabbed something "too hot to handle." As soon as I dropped the pan, I ran to the sink and squeezed the CELLFOOD$^®$ concentrate directly on the burned area. To my amazement, the pain started to diminish right away— and within minutes it was gone. I went back to cooking and didn't think about it again. The next day, one of my weekend guests asked me how the burn was. To my amazement, I had forgotten all about it because there was no blister or pain. There was only a slight red mark where there should have been one of those big, painful water-filled blisters."

RB— Palm Springs, CA

"I was watching a TV broadcast of ABC's 20/20 last night, and the second segment was devoted to the appearance of an especially virulent strain of *E.coli* on fresh vegetables, especially lettuce. Interviews were held with people who became very ill after ingesting what they thought was healthful food. An incident where hundreds of Japanese school children became ill from tain-ted radish sprouts was also reviewed.

In an interview and demonstration with health officials it was shown that even with thorough washing, one or two cells of

E.coli still contaminated the subject lettuce. The conclusion of the program is that our produce is mostly safe, but that we should always be sure to thoroughly wash it before ingesting. After reading the U.S.P. Challenge test given to CELLFOOD®, I saw clearly that CELLFOOD® killed *E.coli* permanently upon contact. If you are concerned by this 20/20 report, I advise simply soaking your fruits and vegetables in a sink full of cold water with about 25-30 drops of CELLFOOD® for about 20 minutes. Then rinse them, bag in plastic, and store in your refrigerator."

SBW— Apple Valley, CA

"I have had much success with CELLFOOD®. I've been handicapped for years due to a medical misdiagnosis by doctors; I was treated for arthritis when I had tuberculosis of the bone. The medicine I was given fused my joints, damaged my entire system, and left me in continuous pain.

The first day I took CELLFOOD® I slept more than I had at any one time in years. After a few days my energy increased to where I now have several more hours each day of active life— and more movement in my joints. I also have used CELLFOOD® topically on both my fingernails and toenails— both of which had fungus and poor circulation. Within days my nails became smoother, and the cuticles became pink and the fungus healed."

JAJ— Torrance, CA

"My life has changed dramatically since I began taking CELL-FOOD® 2 months ago. The effects of taking this product were almost immediate. I have been diagnosed as having Epstein-Barr and have had a major problem with fatigue and well-being for years. For quite a while my work day was limited, and that took all of my energy; I too often had to tell my husband I was too tired to do anything else.

When I started taking CELLFOOD® my energy level tripled within 24 hours. I began to get projects done that had been on the back burner for months. I no longer needed to have caffeine to get me up and around in the morning. Life became so much easier, happier and more full as a result of taking this product.

Now, after just 2 months, I have so much energy that I've started taking dance lessons, am adding more clients to my practice, and my house is cleaner than it's been in years. Every day I thank God for sending me CELLFOOD®."

SK—Sarasota, FL

"I have always had very poor circulation with cold extremities and somewhat blue or grey coloration in my fingers and toes. When I use the CELLFOOD®, my circulation picks up, within minutes my toes and fingers 'pink up,' and there is warmth from the better circulation and oxygen.

In addition, I had the herbicide 2-4D go into my well and it caused severe bowel problems, one of which was constipation. Now that I'm using CELLFOOD®, I no longer take lots of fiber and psyllium husk for the constipation, the problems I formerly had with digestion are gone, and I can eat a greater variety of foods.

I feel a huge increase in energy when using CELLFOOD®— and with that, an increased ability to focus and process thoughts. I've tried many different forms of oxygen, but none that have given me the increase in energy, circulation and focus that CELLFOOD® does. The other plus with CELLFOOD® is that there are not the side effects of the free radicals that I had with other products.

I've used other natural and mined minerals, and taken amino acids and enzyme formulations, all with minimal results. With CELLFOOD® I see results in all these different areas. The CELLFOOD®— even though it's in a small container— lasts me beyond the month and saves me money in the long run because I do not have to buy many of the expensive supplements that I used to buy.

I now am experiencing better health and healing from adding the important and vital trace elements in CELLFOOD®. I highly recommend this product to all of my customers."

MR— Providence, UT

"In late September, 1999, we began using CELLFOOD®. By this time my mother-in-law was in the later stages of Alzheimer's disease. She had been on the pharmaceutical medication Cognex, but had to be taken off of it because of side effects. She had then been on Aricept since February, but no matter what the doctor could give her, she was lethargic and unresponsive. She wouldn't feed herself, and slumped on the couch all day, sleeping.

When we started her on CELLFOOD®, there was a dramatic change. Not only was she awake more, noticing what was going on around her— and talking again— but she became more vigorous, and began walking with some energy. It is wonderful to have her 'present' again."

VM— Bedford, TX

"Our daughter had laser surgery on her back in late November, when we were in Florida. She was taking double doses of CELLFOOD® and a high quality vitamin for two months prior to the surgery. It was a complete success and she was up and walking at home that night. We maintained the regime for two weeks post surgery, then tapered off. I have no doubt that the CELLFOOD® played a major part in the rapid healing process as there was a good deal of irritation in the area surrounding the herniated disc. This collateral damage was causing her great discomfort prior to the surgery and the surgeon said it would take quite a while to heal, but in less than 30 days she was back to normal routines and drove herself back to Atlanta on January 7th. She had formerly been unable to drive more than a few miles without severe back pain. Needless to say, I have only positive things to say about this product, and tell as many people as I can of its potential use in their lives."

CW—Jeddah, Saudi Arabia

"What exactly is CELLFOOD®, you might ask? It is a formulation of clear liquid drops that I firmly believe has saved my mother's life. She is 79 years old, and has been suffering from congestive heart failure and thyroid disease, among her ailments. The diuretics she'd been taking had depleted her electrolytes so severely that she had to be hospitalized for intravenous therapy. In January 2000, her doctor ordered 24-hour oxygen therapy. Her fingers and skin were turning greyish-blue. Her immune system had become very suppressed, and she began suffering from sores in her mouth and on her skin. She was weak, fatigued, losing muscle tone, and was hallucinating, dizzy, disoriented and unable to eat. She was dying before my eyes; the situation seemed hopeless.

Three weeks ago Friday I wandered into the health food store and there sat this miracle bottle of drops. I picked up the information, read it repeatedly— and purchased the product for my mother. The next day my mom called me. She said that within three hours of taking 4 drops of CELLFOOD® in water she somehow felt different, as if she was plugged into a light switch and energized. During the couse of the first week the weakness faded, and she was no longer confused, disoriented or hallucinating. Not only was she able to carry on a conversation, but her need for supplemental oxygen had been decreased to approximately just 2-3 hours per week. Today she is walking, sleeping more soundly, and has a hearty appetite. Topically, I began placing drops on her skin and in her mouth. The sores in her mouth disappeared the same day, and within three days there were no traces of infection, let alone scars. The quality of my mother's life has improved so dramatically in such a short time that she is again looking forward to living, rather than waiting to die.

I have one more testimonial— this one regards myself. Recently, I had a growth removed from my nose. I put a few drops of cellfood on the area after the surgery. One week later when I returned to have the stitches removed, the doctor looked puzzled— and remarked what a fast healer I was. They had never seen a surgical area heal before having the stitches removed. And there is no scar at all remaining now. I can't thank you enough; we have recommended CELLFOOD® to everyone we know."

MA— St. Petersburg, FL

"I have fibromyalgia to the point that every cell in my body hurts. It also causes me to feel tense and constricted all over, and my thinking is slow and foggy.

After taking CELLFOOD® for just 24 hours I could feel more energy, I felt looser, and my thinking became much clearer. Within a month I wondered if I needed the CELLFOOD® because I felt so much better. I briefly stopped, but soon realized that I need to keep taking it. I tell everyone I know with any health problem to try this product."

SH— Grants Pass, OR

Biography of the Author

Dr. David Dyer is a Vietnam veteran and former aircraft commander. He transported troops by helicopter during his tour of duty, and was awarded the Distinguished Flying Cross, Bronze Star and Purple Heart. While serving in Vietnam he was exposed to traditional herbal methods of healing. This began his quest to help others take control of their own health.

Dr. Dyer became more interested in his own health in 1977, when he was experiencing some personal health challenges. He began fasting on a regular basis and encouraged others to do the same— and soon became known among friends as a 'health nut.' Researching cutting-edge ideas about health and well-being became a way of life for him. He consumed books by authors like Dr. Norman Walker and Dr. Paavo Airola— men famous for their outstanding contributions to the world of personal health.

In 1994 he returned to school and became a Licensed Massage Therapist and Licensed Colon Therapist. In 1998 he completed a four-year goal and was awarded a Doctorate in Naturopathy from The Trinity College of Natural Health in Indiana, USA. During those years of study he owned and operated a highly successful health and nutrition center, again helping people understand the importance of taking responsibility for their own health.

Postscript

The frontiers of human healing are continually being expanded, and now at an even faster rate than ever before. Just as this book was ready to go to press I received word of a research study being conducted in South Africa which holds immense promise for the inhabitants of planet earth. More detail will be coming forth— and no doubt will be documented in future updates of this book— but it seems that an 18 month study involving 552 people certified as being HIV+(positive) has shown a 96% success rate in returning their blood test results to negative when using CELLFOOD®. It further appears that those patients who had not previously received chemical medication were the fastest to respond to CELLFOOD® therapy, sometimes reversing their condition in as little as 3 months. It was also reported to me that those who had received chemical medication did sometimes require other additional natural elements in addition to CELLFOOD® and required up to 18 months to respond successfully. We are hopeful of receiving full documentation as soon as possible concerning this extremely hopeful news.

— Dr. David S. Dyer